ALL ABOUT TOBACCO

2nd edition

I0416032

BY
KIBOKO FRANÇOISE MACHOZI

www.savelife.co.za

CONTENTS

HISTORY AND ORIGINS OF TOBACCO

Tobacco refers to the more than seventy plant species within the genus *Nicotiana* of the nightshade family.

This plant takes its origins from Tobago Island in South America.

Indians living there were the first to know and use the plant.

Its psychological and medical effects made it easier to trade, and it did not delay becoming known worldwide, starting in France.

Christopher Columbus brought the plant from America to Spain and Portugal.

In Spain tobacco was used as a flower or garden plant until the family doctor of the Spanish king Philip II promoted it to a medicine.

In 1559 Jean Nicot, French ambassador to Portugal, sent the plant to the French queen Catherine de' Medici, who used it to treat the migraines of her son François II. Later biochemists discovered the active ingredient responsible for the psychological and medical effects and named it after the French ambassador Jean Nicot.

This is the origin of the name *Nicotiana tabacum*.

Tobacco contributed to the economic development of the southern United States of America.

Tobacco is smoked by ± 1.1 billion people, which is ± one-third of adults worldwide, and causes 5.4 million deaths per year.

In developed countries the number of tobacco smokers decreases while in developing countries it increases by 34 percent every year.

TOBACCO AGRICULTURE

Tobacco plants may grow under any climatic condition, but hot weather is much more suitable for them to grow.

In cold weather the plant takes 150 days before it may be used, while in hot weather it only takes sixty days.

Tobacco agriculture is not recommended in chloride-rich soil, but it is recommended to put plants in potassium-rich soil.

For good results the soil must be a bit moist and well ventilated.

To prevent tobacco seeds from being eaten by insects, it is sown in cold frames, and after it is transplanted into the soil.

The harvest is made by hand, and it is stored to allow slow oxidation.

Tobacco is consumed by smoking, sniffing, chewing, and dipping it.

It may also be used as an ingredient in some medicines; it may be used as a pesticide agent as well.

COMPOSITION OF TOBACCO SMOKE

Tobacco smoke may be divided into gaze and particles.

Tobacco smoke has about four thousand particles, including the following:

1. Nicotine

2. Carbon monoxide

3. Irritants:

- Ammonia
- Volatile nitrosamine
- Hydrogen
- Cyanide
- Sulfur compounds (H2S, COS, CS2, SO2)
- Hydrocarbon
- Alcohol
- Aldehydes
- Ketone

Some of these irritants inhibit ciliary activity in human lungs.

4. Tar is a common term used to identify all the carcinogens found in tobacco smoke.

It is sticky, brown, and has the ability to stain teeth, fingernails, and lung tissues.

Some tar elements:
- Carcinogen benzo (a) pyrene
- Hydrogen cyanide
- Free radicals
- Metals
- Radioactive compounds

NICOTINE

Nicotine is a colorless volatile alkaloid found in tobacco leaves.

It constitutes 0.2 to 5 percent of the weight of dry tobacco leaves.

Nicotine reaches your brain eight to ten seconds after you have inhaled tobacco smoke, and its traces are found everywhere in the body, even in breast milk.

NICOTINE SIDE EFFECTS

Nervous system

Nicotine stimulates the central and peripheral nervous system and is responsible for addiction.

In lower dosages, nicotine makes you to relax and feel good, but the greater the dose the more dangerous it becomes, possibly leading to a fit, generalized stroke, or coma.

Nicotine causes nervousness, sleeplessness, anxiety, abnormal dreams, dizziness, sweating, and weakness.

It increases respiratory movement by stimulating the respiratory center found in the brain.

Respiratory system

Nicotine stimulates bronchial secretions, and this process leads to chronic obstructive pulmonary disease.

Circulatory system

Nicotine increases the oxygen requirement of the heart muscle but decreases the supply of oxygen.

Nicotine constricts peripheral blood vessels, raises blood pressure, and accelerates heart beating.

Nicotine damages the lining inside blood vessels.

Nicotine lowers the level of good cholesterol (HDL) and increases free fatty acids, and all of this contributes to heart attack.

Nicotine increases the risk of developing thromboses.

Digestive system

Nicotine increases salivary secretion, inhibits hunger, and causes nausea, vomiting, and diarrhea. Nicotine causes insulin resistance characterized by an increased level of sugar in the blood and a dry mouth.

Musculoskeletal system

Nicotine causes joint pain and muscle pain.

Urinary system

Nicotine decreases urinary flow.

Skin

On the skin nicotine causes rashes.

Other nicotine effects

Nicotine also causes swelling of the face and mouth.

CARBON MONOXIDE SIDE EFFECTS

Carbon monoxide is a colorless, odorless, and tasteless tobacco particle that binds itself to hemoglobin and inhibits its oxygen transportation. This situation leads to hypoxia.

IRRITANTS' SIDE EFFECTS

The irritants found in tobacco smoke provoke irritation inside the lungs, inhibit ciliary movement, and are responsible for the chronic bronchitis noticed by many smokers.

TAR ELEMENTS' SIDE EFFECTS

Carcinogen benzo (a) pyrene, which fixes itself to the cells of airways and to the cells of different organs in the human body, leads to tumor development.

Lungs have tiny hairs called cilia that move out foreign bodies from the lungs. Hydrogen cyanide stops cilia activity. As a result, all poisonous elements found in tobacco can build up and damage the lungs.

Free radicals may damage the heart and blood vessels. Together with bad cholesterol (LDL), they build up fat on the arterial walls. This can lead to heart disease, stroke, hypertension, and aneurism.

Tobacco smoke has metals that are dangerous, including cadmium, arsenic, and lead. Some of these are carcinogenic.

Radioactive compounds are carcinogenic.

TOBACCO'S EFFECTS ON THE BODY'S ORGANS

In the lungs tobacco causes irritation, narrowing of airways, and excessive mucus production, all of which can lead to chronic obstructive lung disease, which is characterized by shortness of breath and chronic cough.

ON THE CIRCULATORY SYSTEM

In the circulatory system tobacco does the following:

- Raises blood pressure.
- Constricts blood vessels in the skin. This condition is responsible for hypothermia noticed among smokers.
- Decreases oxygenation of cells.
- Creates stickier blood that is predisposed to clotting.
- Damages the lining inside the arteries, which contributes to atherosclerosis.
- Decreases blood circulation to the extremities.
- Increases the risk of heart attack and stroke.

ON THE DIGESTIVE SYSTEM

In the digestive tract, tobacco irritants cause ulcers and accelerate peristaltic movement; this is the reason why smokers go to the toilet after their first cigarette in the morning.

Tobacco promotes gingivitis, decreases the ability to taste, causes gastritis, and increases ulcer pain.

In the liver tobacco increases bile secretion, which contributes to the laxative effect of the first cigarette in the morning.

In the pancreas tobacco decreases pancreatic secretion; as a consequence, the acid level increases in the first part of the small intestine and causes peptic ulcers.

ON THE MUSCULOSKELTAL SYSTEM

In the musculoskeletal system, tobacco causes the tightening of some muscles and decreases bone density.

ON THE SKIN

Tobacco damages the same protein that is damaged in Werner syndrome (genetic disorder characterized by premature aging) and causes premature wrinkles.

Tobacco use places you in the presence of life-threatening fire.

Tobacco use also causes a loss of sensitivity on the fingers.

ON TEETH

Tobacco changes the normal appearance of teeth and gives them a dark yellowish color.

ON THE IMMUNE SYSTEM

Tobacco use decreases the capacity of the body to fight against disease.

ON SEX

Tobacco affects your sexual life as well and may also affect your fecundity.

ON PREGNANCY

Tobacco use can affect both mother and child during pregnancy:

To the mother

- Miscarriage
- Premature delivery
- Stillborn
- Premature rupture of membranes
- Insertion of placenta at the wrong place (placenta previa)

To the baby

- Low birth weight
- Sudden infant death syndrome
- Mental retardation
- Diabètes mellitus
- Obesity

DISEASES CAUSED BY TOBACCO

The following diseases can be the result of tobacco use:

- Heart attack and coronary disease
- Stroke
- Chronic obstructive pulmonary disease
- Emphysema (presence of pus in lungs tissues)
- Lung cancer, larynx cancer, laryngeal polyps, mouth cancer, throat cancer, esophageal cancer, stomach cancer, colorectal cancer, and pancreatic cancer
- Ulcers

Did you know that half of smokers die of tobacco-threatening diseases and that they die ten years earlier than nonsmokers?

The risk of cancer depends on several factors:

- Amount of tobacco consumed on a daily basis
- Age at which a person starts smoking
- Form in which tobacco is taken
- Duration of smoke inhalation

What can be done to help people stop smoking?

- Stop tobacco advertisements
- Increase taxes for tobacco importation
- Campaign against tobacco at schools and workplaces and on radio and television
- Limit the number of tobacco stores

TOBACCO CESSATION METHODS

The following ten cessation methods can help you reduce or stop your tobacco use.

1. Cold turkey method

This method involves a sudden and total cessation of tobacco.

The percentage rate of failure is higher.

2. Gradual reduction

This method involves gradually decreasing your daily dose of tobacco until total cessation.

3. Hypnosis

This method involves putting an individual to sleep through hypnosis, whereby he or she then becomes able to accept suggestions of the hypnotist to quit tobacco use.

For better results hypnosis must not be used alone but in association with another method like nicotine replacement.

The percentage of success is evaluated at 65 percent.

4. Sophrology

Without a person knowing, usually before sleeping, the master makes him or her listen to a CD that talks about the bad side effects of tobacco.

5. Nicotine replacement

This method gives you gradual lower doses of nicotine to help you to cope with nicotine dependency until you stop completely.

It gives you nicotine without tar or any tobacco elements.

It helps you to decrease gradually your cravings for cigarettes and the withdrawal syndrome.

There are many nicotine replacement products: gums, lozenges, nasal sprays, inhalators, lollipops, and patches.

Patches gradually release a small amount of nicotine in your bloodstream. This product is good for people who smoke all throughout the day but may not respond quickly to a craving.

Gums, lozenges, nasal sprays, inhalators, and lollipops give you a high dose of nicotine at once and help you respond more quickly to a craving.
These products are suitable for people who are smoking only when they have stress or a craving.
You may find some of these nicotine replacement products in pharmacies or some supermarkets.

Many pharmacies or supermarkets that supply nicotine replacements also have support teams for helping smokers stop smoking.

6. Ziban

This is an anti-smoking pill that reduces nicotine withdrawal syndrome.

It does not contain nicotine, but it seems to have effects similar to nicotine.

7. Chantix

Chantix ou varenicline tartrate ou champix for Europeans is a partial agonist of the nicotine receptor.

8. Low-level laser therapy

This method is similar to acupuncture.

Low-level laser therapy is oriented to the face, hands, and wrists to stimulate the brain to release a large amount of endorphins in order to prevent nicotine withdrawal syndrome.

What are endorphins?

Endorphins are natural chemicals produced by your body to release stress and to increase energy.

9. Acupuncture

This Chinese method of healing is also successful.

The process consists of inserting a very thin needle into a specific area of the body to stimulate a natural healing response. It stimulates your body to produce endorphins.

10. Electronic cigarette or E-cigarette

The electronic cigarette is a recent and powerful method for tobacco cessation.

Eighty-nine percent of smokers quit smoking using this method.

One cartridge of an E-cigarette gives you 16 mg of tobacco, which is equivalent to thirty normal or traditional cigarettes but without tar, odor, flame, or any carcinogen.

There are E-cigarettes without tobacco but with 16 mg of menthol.

A kit of E-cigarettes contains the following:

- One cartridge
- One rechargeable battery
- One USB charger

CONCLUSION

It is easier to start a bad pattern than to stop it.
If you are not a smoker, it is better never to be one of them, but if you are smoking there is a way to stop.

If there is only one person who manages to stop smoking, you may be the second one.

Nothing is impossible, as life is a matter of decision.

Never forget that good decisions impact your life in positive ways and bad decisions impact it in negative ways.

My prayer is that you do understand this message and make a good decision.

GOLDEN ADVICE: SSEE

Stop smoking
Stop drinking alcohol
Eat healthy
Exercise

BIBLIOGRAPHY

FT, Le groupe France Tabac, *l'histoire du tabac* Buxidanicophiles sur le tabatieres snuffboxes, le site des amteurs et collectionneurs de tabatieres, *L'origine du tabac*

Doctssimo, Arreter de fumer, *l'histoire du tabac* J. Courtejoie, dictionnaire medical pour les regions tropicales, 1983, DRC

Dr E.G. Peeters, *Le cancer* MV bibliotheque,117 Marabout universite, Nº 66/49

Andres Dufour, Maud Cousin, Philippe Augendre, *cesser de fumer*, edition77190Damarie lesLys,1975

Revue *Developpement et Sante* Nº 26, Imprimerie Magenta RC 309257137, 1980

Directrice Van Hand Boww Bossen Veetelt, *Bulletin Agricole du Congo Belge* 1953

Croquet Htier, *Production du prince et methode*, 2eme edition, 1961

Tabazaire 50 ans, *Programme des manifestation du 50eme anniversaire de la SZ AKL, Tabazaire* 1989 *Renseignement sur les drogues, foundation of Ontario*, 1989

Reactions anormales a la drogue, publication autorisee par ministre de la sante et bien etre sociale, Canada, 1978

Dr Onyembe PML, *Environnement et industrie du tabac*

Revue soins, *Pathologie du tabac,* Tome 25, Nº 11, 05 juin 1980

Sante du monde Nº 525,Juin 1989

Sante medecine, *la cigarette et ses substances nocives*

Science avenir, sante, *Tabac : La liste des 93 produits toxiques de la fumee de cigarette.*

Sante chez nous, *Tabagisme, La composition de la fumee*

Arreterfumer.fr, *Les effets du tabac sur les poumons*

Santemedecine.net, *Effets du tabac sur la sante*

Arreter de fumer, *Les effets du tabac sur les poumons d'un fumeur*

Doctissimo, *Arreter de fumer, Tabac : garre aux maladies du cœur*
e-sante.be, *Guide prevention du risque cardiovasculaire, une cigarette en plein cœur*

Universite de Liege, *Effets des differents composes du tabac.*

La therapie cognitivo-comportementale : *Efficace contre l'addiction au tabac,* www.arret-tabac-bienfait.com/la-therapie....

Arreter de fumer, www.doctissimo.fr/thm/dossiers/tab.

Cigarette electronique, www.wikipedia.org/wiki/cigarette_%25

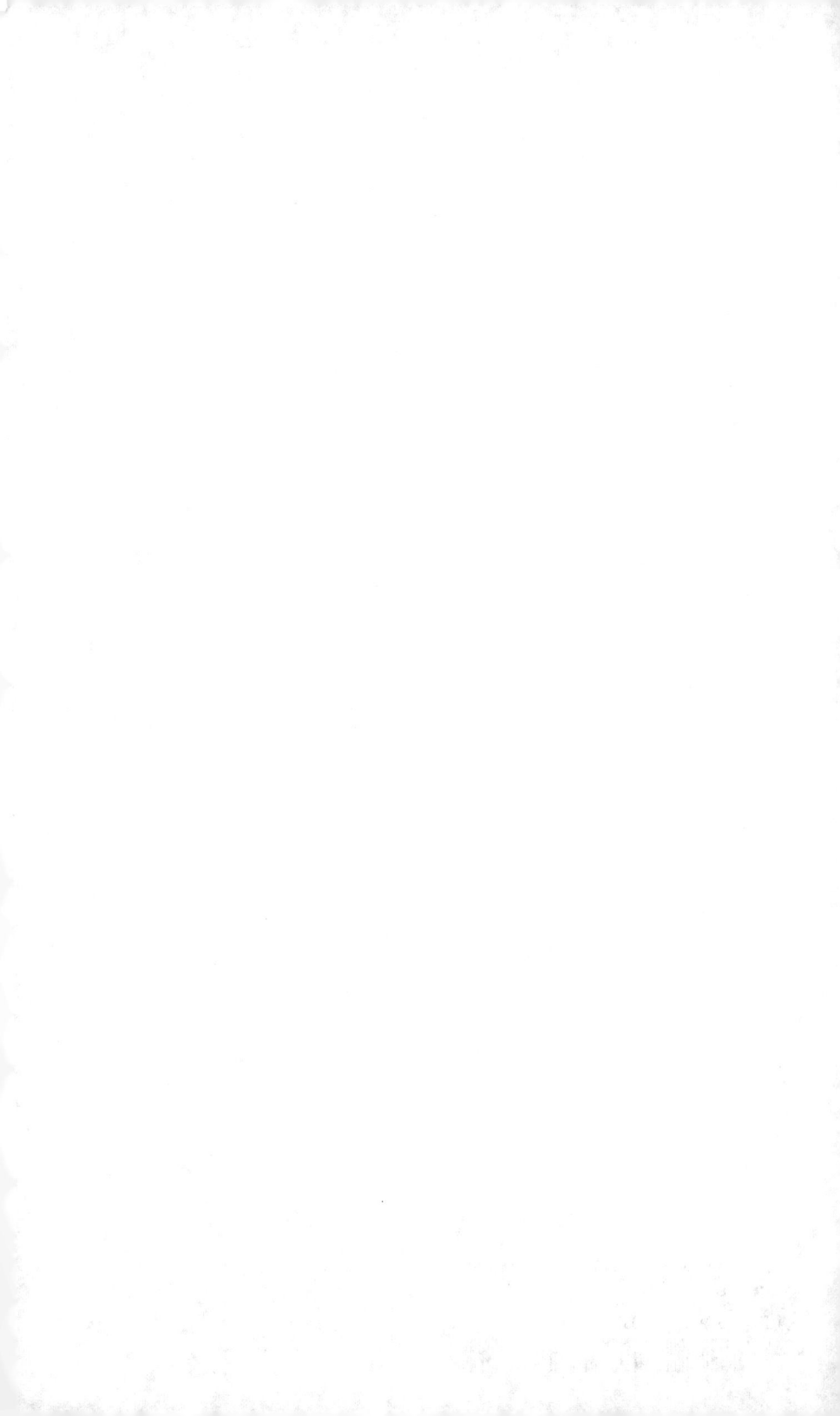